Kitchen Safety

Tips to Prevent Kitchen Accidents

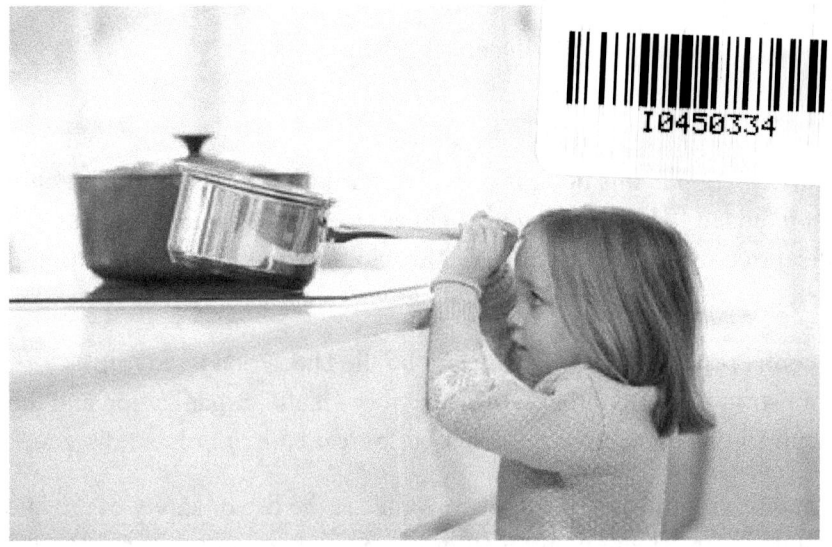

Disaster Management Series

Dueep J. Singh

Mendon Cottage Books

JD-Biz Publishing

Check out some of the other Healthy Gardening Series books at Amazon.com

Gardening Series on Amazon

Check out some of the other Health Learning Series books at Amazon.com

Health Learning Series on Amazon

Table of Contents

Introduction

Did you know that around 600 people, in the USA alone, die annually due to fires caused in kitchens? This is a global problem, especially where fires are allowed to reign supreme, because people do not know how to control them or even how to prevent them.

Kitchen accidents are not restricted to the kitchen alone. They can occur when you are cooking outdoors, especially during barbecues.

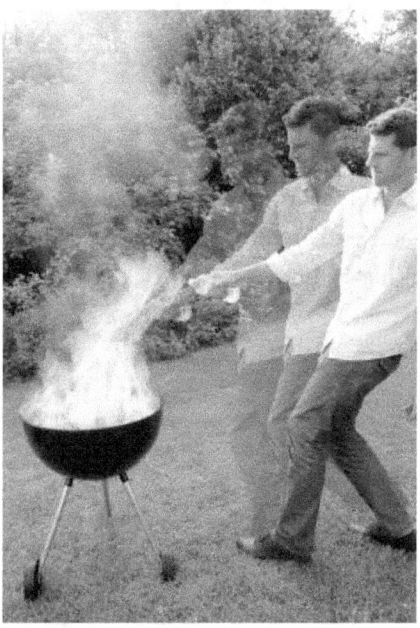

A little bit of care taken while barbecuing could have prevented possibly serious burns.

Remember that your kitchen is an accident zone, like the rest of your house. So a little bit of common sense used right now is going to prevent accidents from happening.

Burn Injuries While Cooking

If you are fond of cooking in the kitchen, it is possible that you have faced burn injuries, sometime or the other. These can either be mild burn injuries or they could have been serious burns. And all these injuries could have been easily been avoided if you had just use some elementary precautions.

Hot Fat

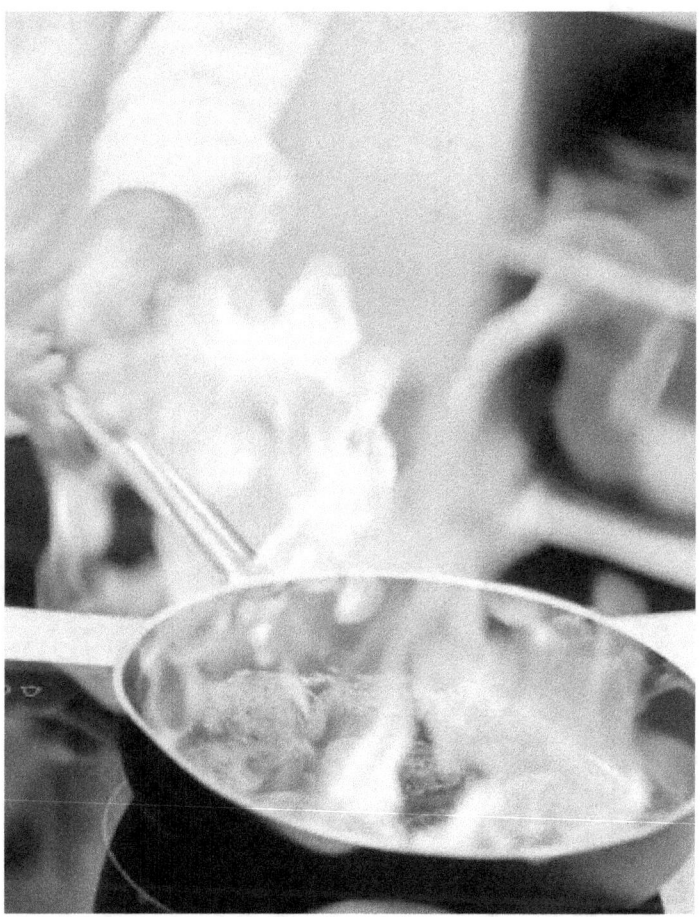

Never allow the oil to heat so much that it catches fire.

No one should be alone when they are using deep fat for frying. Especially when this is the first time you are trying out your deep fat frying techniques in a wok over high heat. Do not try it out yourself, and for the first time, if you are an amateur in the cooking field. Just look at an experienced cook and see the way he/she handles deep frying.

Hot fat has a tendency to splash. Some cooks are so used to having miniscule droplets of hot fat, sprinkling them, that they do not mind being in close proximity to a hot frying pan while cooking. This is definitely not a very pleasant experience for a person who is being exposed to deep frying techniques for the first time. So make sure that your face and body is well away from a heart frying pan, when you are dealing with hot fat.

Water in Fat

I was watching one of my friends cooking and I saw her wash the frying pan, and place it on the heat without allowing it to dry. After that she put in a teaspoonful of oil. When I told her that the water droplets would begin to sizzle in the fat and splutter as the oil heated up, she just shrugged her shoulders.

I got out of the kitchen fast. She was just an accident waiting to happen. So that is why if you want to fry anything, especially by heating fat first, make sure that the saucepan or the frying pan is completely dry.

Water or any other liquid dropped into hot fat – whether it is deep or shallow – is going to sizzle and splutter. The hotter the fat, the more violently the tiny droplets of fat will be thrown into the air. They are going to burn any available surface, including the skin of your exposed face and hands.

Also, remember to switch off the burner, before you put in any liquid into hot fat. Tomatoes, sausages, and even roe have this tendency to splutter the moment they come in contact with hot fat. Once these items are in your skillet, and have "simmered down" you can turn the flame on again. Stand well back and cover with a lid or plate when possible.

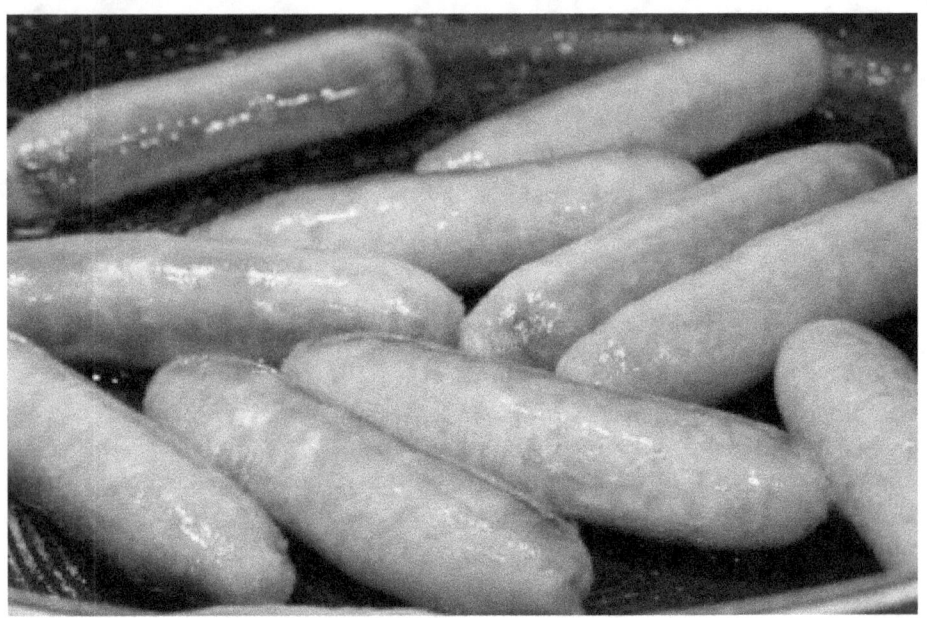

Do not put sausages in a fry pan, full of heated fat, without switching off the flame beforehand. When they stop sizzling, you can light the flame again.

Steam Accidents

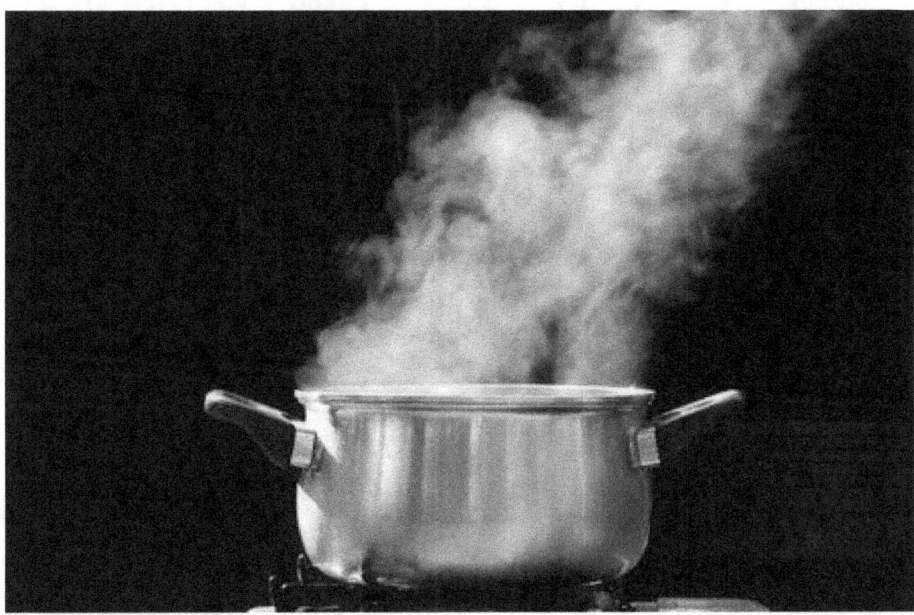

Now steam is one of the most powerful of accident causing factors in your kitchen. Steam is just hot liquid turned into air. You are not going to touch boiling hot water, are you? So why would you want to expose your hand or your face to steam, which just happens to be boiling water in gaseous form?

Remember that steam is powerful enough to cause as bad a burn as would hot water, when it falls on your skin. It is going to scald the skin.

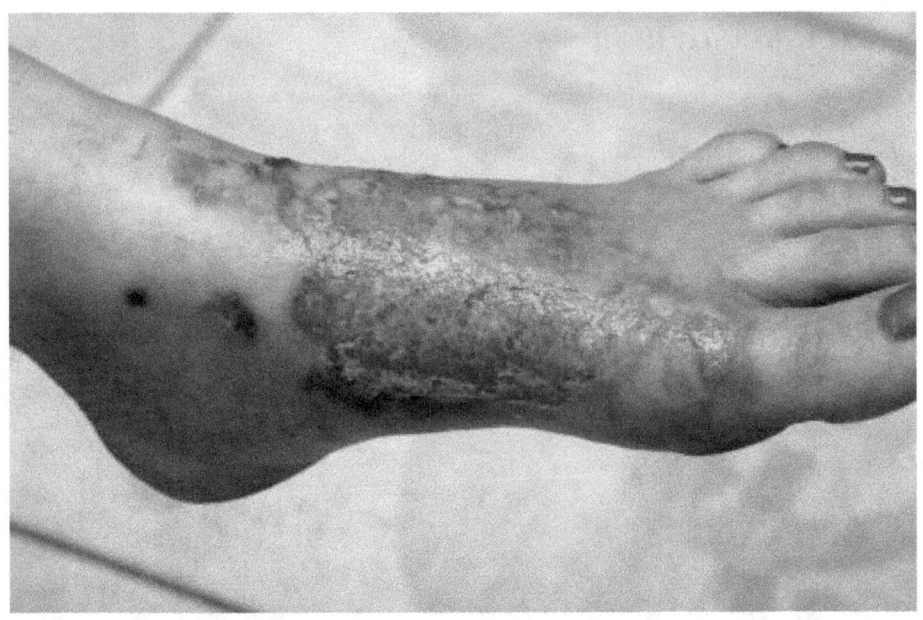

A steam burn is going to be as painful as any other burn.

Spilt Saucepans

This may sound unusual, but most of the accidents causing the kitchen are due to hot food cooking in saucepans being spilled accidentally. This is going to happen when the handle comes off. It may also happen if the handle is "jutting out," when on the cooking range and you knock over the saucepan by accident, when in passing.

The saucepan may then be thrown off balance and spill all the hot liquid over you or over anybody else in the vicinity.

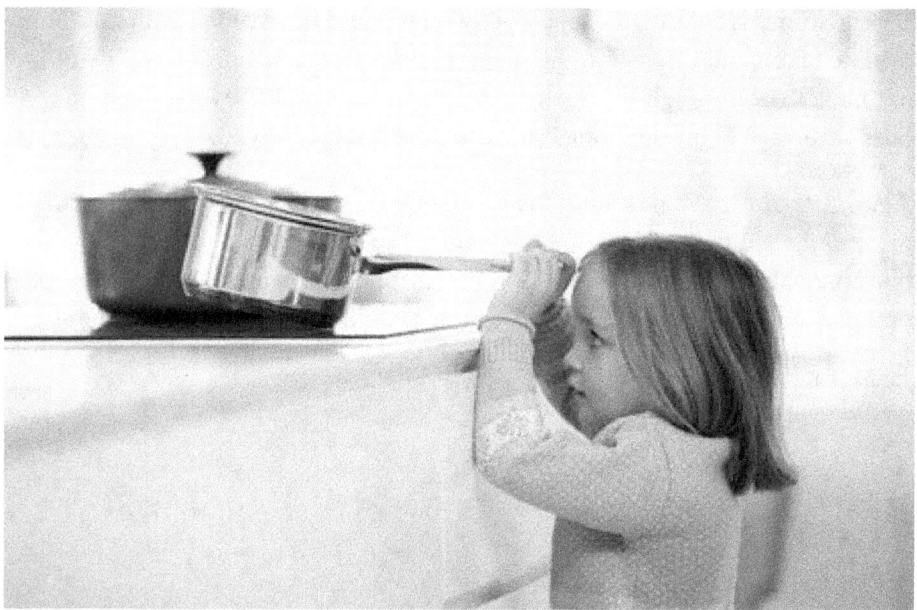

This little girl is risking an accident by handling a hot pan, without any adult in the vicinity.

I remember to do a 3 monthly inspection of all the handles of my cooking utensils, including frying pans, saucepans and pressure cookers. And also if I have a feeling that one of the fastening screws has come adrift, and the handle is loose.

That is because you cannot afford to take a chance that you may be left with just the handle in your hand and an overfilled hot saucepan cascading all over the kitchen counters or even over you.

That happened to me once. The handle of a skillet was loose, – I had lost some fastening screws – but I knew that the plastic handle had been inserted in a metal handle attached to the skillet in which the screws were fastened. So I was just taking the sausages off, when suddenly the handle broke into two and down went the saucepan, breaking a plate, while I managed to jump away from the hot fat. 2 of my toes, however, got burnt.

So due to my stupidity, this accident which could be avoided with a little bit of time taken and effort to tighten and replace two missing screws, I would not have to go through the agony of burnt toes. And believe you me, fat burns are very painful. Do not allow that to happen to you.

Also, be careful when turning the handles inward for safety, not to leave them extended over a flame or hot plate. The handle may get hot enough to burn the palm of your hand badly if it is gripped unawares. Never use a pan or a part with a handle, which is loose or which turns the moment you grip it.

Hot Dishes

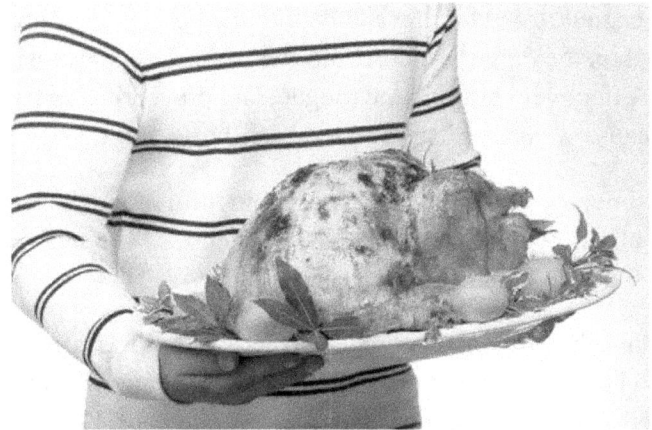

This looks delicious, but taking it out of the oven would have been a very careful affair. And also, care would have been taken while transferring the roast from the hot cooking pan to the serving dish.

Remember that when you are taking out something from the oven, especially when you are reaching to the back of the oven where you just put in the potatoes on to bake, be careful not to let your forearms touch the hot racks. This may not be a serious burn, but it is going to be painful.

Make sure you use mitts when removing a hot dish from an oven or from the microwave.

Dish Testing Dish Testing – 1… 2… 3

Many of us cannot resist dipping a ladle into the hot tempting aromatic soup being cooked on the range. And because we are impatient, in it goes into our mouths, effectively burning the tongue, and preventing us from enjoying the soup because we have blisters on our poor burnt tongue.

So the next time you are tempted to taste a spoonful of any hot soup, sauce or anything else for seasoning – that is your excuse… – remember to blow hard on the spoon to cool it.

That is because the liquid is likely to be exactly at boiling point. This is naturally too hot for the human mouth. Never put anything that has been frying, directly into the mouth before allowing it to cool.

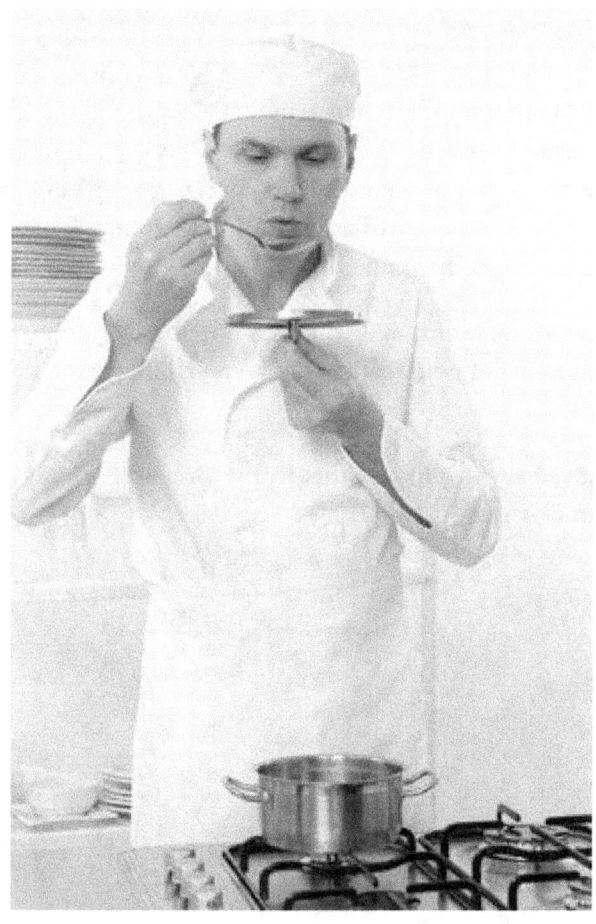

**Now that is sensible. He can have as many spoonfuls of cooled soup as
he likes, before he dishes it up.**

Fire in the Kitchen

One of the most common of kitchen accidents is a fire in the kitchen because the fat caught fire. If the fat is really a very small quantity, a mere film of shallow fat on the bottom of the frying pan, keep calm, stand well back and wait for it to go out which it is going to do in a few moments. Remember to switch off the flame.

If it is more serious than this, and if it does not go out quickly or if it sets fire to anything else, get help from some responsible person or call for the Fire Service.

You should never try to put out this fire with water. That is going to be a disaster of major proportions.

Treating Fire Burns

Tiny burns can usually be effectively treated with burn jelly or burn creams. These are over the counter remedies which are normally found at your nearest drugstore.

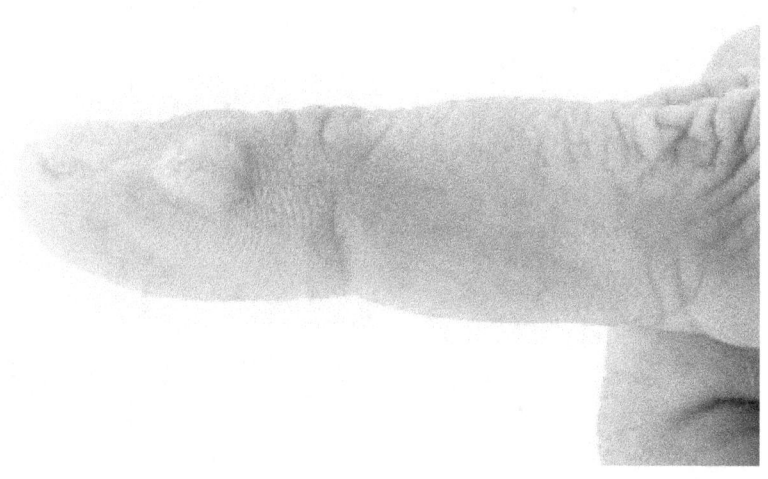

Prevent blisters from occurring by placing the burnt part under cold water. If blisters do occur, puncture them with a sterilized needle, dip in antiseptic, and leave **unbandaged. The skin over the wound is going to help heal it faster.**

However, if there is no skin over the burn and it is red and raw, call a doctor immediately. That is a serious burn.

Do not put oil on the burns, as is usual in many parts of the world. I normally keep a jar full of honey in the kitchen, and the moment I get burnt – which, alas, is quite often – I just dip a spoon in the honey and spread it on the burn. My job is to cool down the skin. And if I have some row potatoes right at hand, I just slice them and place them on the burns.

You can also dip that affected area in ice cold water. That is going to prevent that skin from blistering.

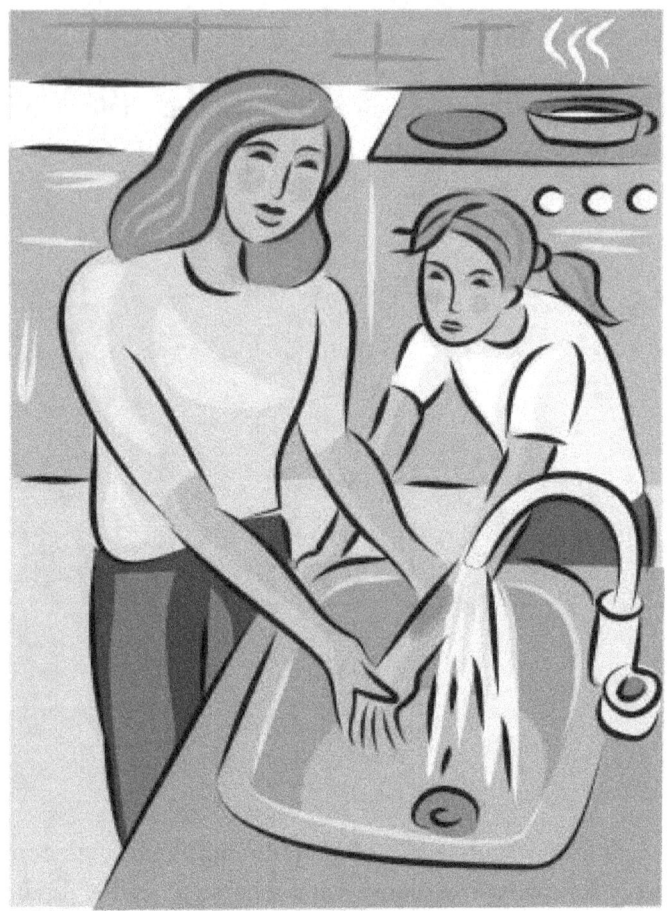

Anything more than a tiny burn should be covered with a clean, dry dressing of linen or gauze and **nothing else**.

If the burn is really bad, the injured person should be made warm and comfortable, and you should call a doctor immediately. Do not neglect the burn, because that area is going to be very vulnerable and prone to infection.

If it is not quite as bad as all that, cover the burn and go to the doctor or the outpatients department of your local hospital and get it treated.

Natural remedies To Treat Burns

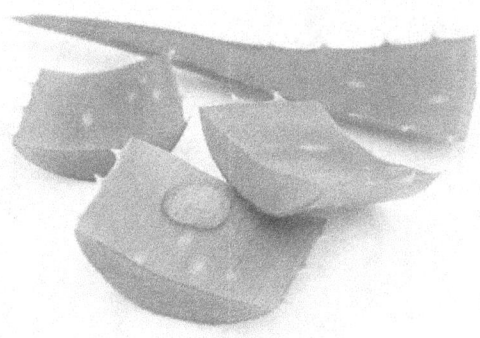

If you have access to Aloe Vera, especially when it is growing in your herb area on the sunny kitchen window sill, just break off a leaf, and apply the inner gel on the burn. This is going to soothe, heal and rejuvenate the affected area. Even serious burns were treated in ancient times with aloe Vera with little scarring.

The moment you burn yourself, the first thing to do is to remove as much heat as possible from the burn, like was done by dipping in that affected area in ice water. You can also hold it in cold water or against an ice pack. If you do not have an icepack around, just take a bag of frozen vegetables. That will serve you as well.

To make sure that the burn heals quickly and well, apply some neat lavender oil, honey, butter, or even marigold cream.

Marigold Cream

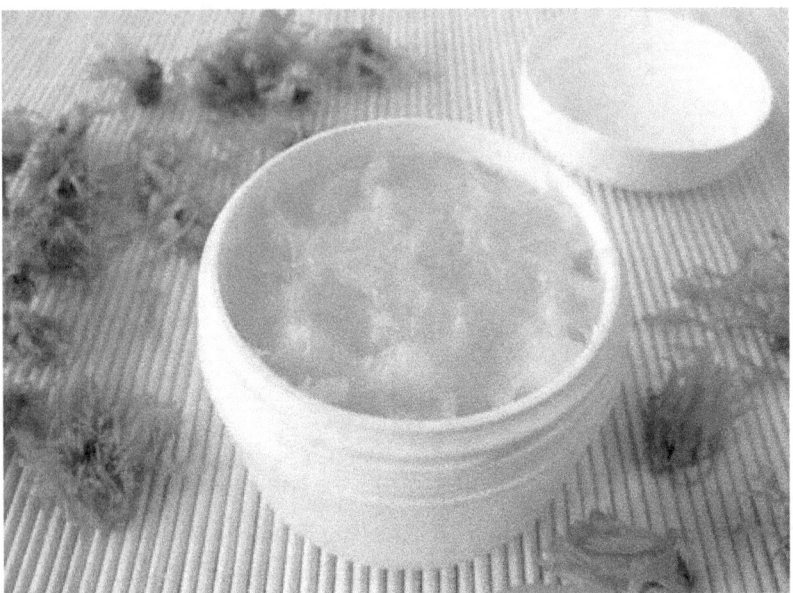

Not only is this an excellent skin cream, but it is the best antiseptic cream for cuts, wounds and bruises.

You can either use Marigold essential oils or you can use fresh Marigold petals to make this exotic, natural skincare cream. Believe you me, this cream can keep you looking youthful, and because it has no chemical preservatives and it is completely natural, it is the much better to a much-hyped, very expensive and branded chemical beauty product out there with chemical-based products like parabens, Ubiquinone , Retinyl Palmitate, Cetearyl Olivate and Sorbitan Olivate in them.

Also, if you use this on cuts and bruises, it is not going to scar the surface, and you are going to have silky smooth skin

Remember that the base for every good rejuvenating skin cream is almond oil and beeswax. Their proportions depend on how creamy or how thick you want the cream to be. Too much of oil will make your cream rather "watery"and too much beeswax will make it solid and chunky.

Melt the beeswax and the almond oil together in a pan placed in another pan with hot water. Once I could not find beeswax easily available in the market, so I used coconut oil, because after all, I was using this homemade cream on my own skin. Also, I placed this cream in the fridge so that I did not have to add a preservative, which you can do further on in the recipe.

Next step – boil the Marigold   petals in 1 cup of water. You may strain it. Now slowly and steadily add the boiled water – petal mixture to the beeswax and almond oil mixture while whisking it thoroughly. Let the emulsifying process takes place slowly.

Just imagine that you are making mayonnaise, when the emulsifying oil is added, drop by drop to the eggs and mustard while whisking. The same process works here. When everything is of a required creamy consistency, you can add the preservatives. Well, I never do that, but you would want to.

Add the preserving chemicals – Sodium benzoate and lactic acid at a ratio of 20 mls lactic acid to 5g sodium benzoate (1/2 tsp). These are readily available at a chemists or a drugstore.

I went a bit further, I chopped up fresh Marigold, rose and jasmine petals finely and added them to my calendula cream to give just that hint of exotic natural fragrance and daintiness. Do you know that this cream is wonderful for skincare as well as for cuts, stings and burns too?

Apart from a vinegar and brown paper poultice, you can treat sprains by using a crushed cabbage leaf on that affected area and leave on until the swelling is reduced.

Then rub in some oil with a little bit of cayenne added to it, to restore the circulation and speed the healing process. This oil is a "hot" oil, thanks to the cayenne. You need to use just a little quantity of oil, because cayenne on your skin is going to burn. Nevertheless, it helps in speeding up the blood supply to that particular area.

Vinegar and Brown Paper Poultice

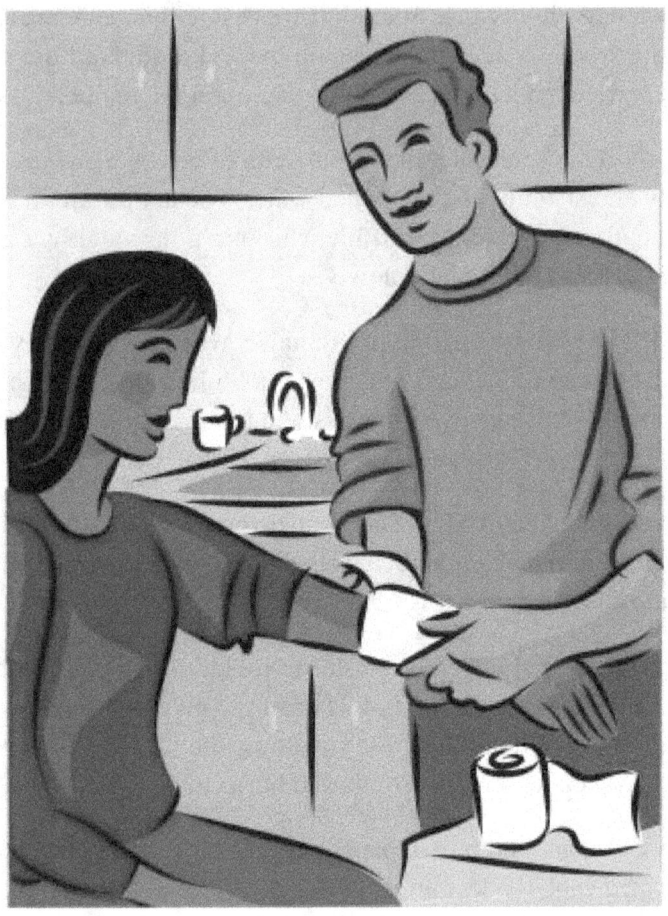

Remember the Jack and Jill nursery rhyme, where Jack fell down and broke his crown and was treated with vinegar and brown paper? That is right, vinegar, in a diluted form is quite efficient to cure cuts and burns.

Cover the injured area with a cotton cloth, which has been soaked in diluted vinegar. This vinegar compress can be used as often as possible, especially when the burn starts to "smart" again.

The best way in which you can treat a bruise – the ancient way – is to make a poultice of vinegar and brown paper.

Put 6 sheets of strong brown paper in a pan and cover with vinegar. Use any good vinegar, as long as it is natural and organic. Here, I am using Sage vinegar because it is extremely good for bruises. This helps in cooling and reducing the swelling.

I make Sage vinegar by bruising more fresh sage leaves by flattening them with a rolling pin, without tearing or breaking them.

After that, put the sage leaves in a pan and just cover with vinegar. Simmer gently for 5 minutes over a very low heat. The vinegar should not boil, but it should steam so that the sage leaves soften and blanch.

Now this Sage vinegar is going to be used to make a brown paper poultice. The vinegar and brown paper in the pan should be steamed over a very low heat for a few minutes. The time is going to depend on the type of paper used.

It should soften and absorb some vinegar without breaking or disintegrating.

Take out the paper and wrap it in overlapping layers around the affected part.Use it as hot as possible and build up several layers. After that, cover with a plastic wrap or cling film.

Bandage tightly. Leave on for 4 hours. You may want to reapply twice a day until the bruising and swelling has subsided.

Normally, I do not go to a hospital, because did you know that in the USA alone, it has been scientifically proven that 5% of the patients going to hospitals caught infections from hospitals and thus added to believe it or not 2,000,000 more patients. [Yes, 6 zeros.] I was shocked when I saw the statistics. So remember that prevention is better than cure. Keep safe in your kitchen, and make sure that you do not do anything which may need you to go to the hospital.

This includes –

Slips and Falls in the Kitchen

Slips, especially in the kitchen can be potentially serious, so wipe up, without a seconds delay, any water or grease that is spilt on the kitchen floor. A greasy floor is more dangerous than a water spill. Besides, that grease on the floor is almost the best way in which you can accumulate lots of grime and dirt, thus adding to the unhygienic and unsafe quotient in your kitchen.

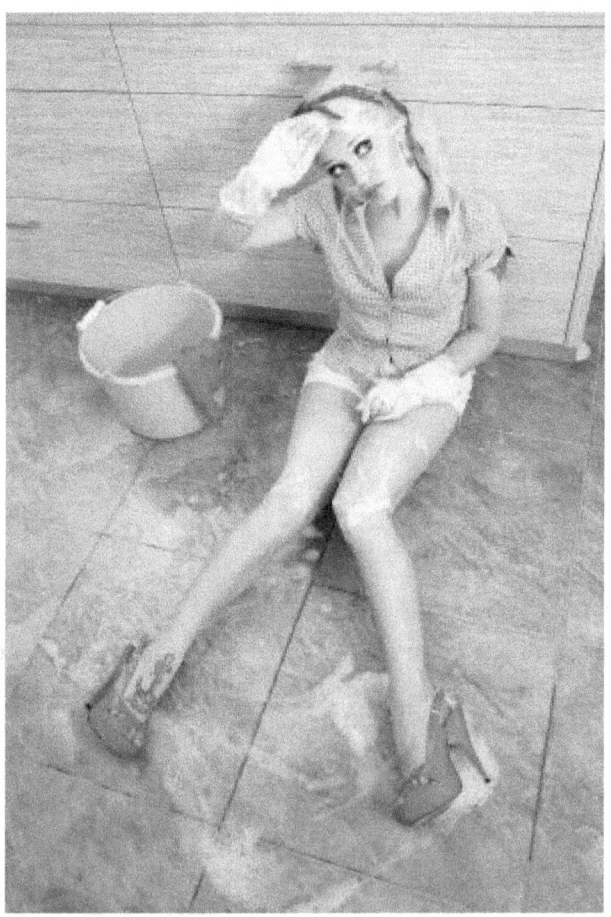

All right, so you are tired of scrubbing the floor, but wipe it clean and dry, before you take a rest break!

Climbing – when you need to climb to a high shelf, to get the provisions stored away there, make sure that there is somebody around you who is holding the ladder firmly. Do not try any of these climbing stunts on your own. Ladders have this nice habit of slipping and sliding away, especially the floor is greasy.

I remember this accident happening when I was a child. My parents were away on an official tour abroad for a month and we children– I was 6 and my younger brother was 3 – were under the care of my grandmother and my uncle.

Uncle had gone to the market to buy some fruit and vegetables. And grandma told us to hold our kitchen ladder, as she climbed up some rungs to get to some stores kept on a higher shelf. We did, to the best of our abilities, but even then, the ladder slipped and grandma fell down.

I still remember the moments of sheer terror, when we two little children stood there horrified, as she lay unconscious on the ground with her head bleeding from a shallow cut. We did not know what to do.

We could not even shout for help, because adults were always around to manage things and children did not have to face that sort of situation in our world ever. Besides, we did not know how to call for help! At that time, children were brought up, wrapped in cotton wool, away from the harsh realities of real life.

Luckily uncle came back really soon and took her to the hospital. And grandma came back within the hour – with her head bandaged, because luckily, she had not fallen far and had not suffered from any concussion or bad aftereffects – to reassure us, and everything was right in our world again.

But that incident has made me very wary of climbing up any stepladders, anytime, anywhere. You could call it a phobia! Nevertheless, remember that when you have to climb up a step ladder, have an adult around. At least he can ring for help, if the ladder slips.

Instead of ladders, I would prefer standing on strong, steady chairs or using proper kitchen steps which are steadier. But even then a steady and strong adult hand should be around to hold the chair or the kitchen steps firmly.

Jumping, climbing and using chair arms or wobbly stools for this purpose are surefire shortcuts to the hospital.

Items Stored on Higher Shelves

I remember another friend of mine – yes, most of us humans are accident prone, due to sheer carelessness – jumping up to get some tins of a higher shelf. She accidentally knocked down more tins than were needed – luckily not on her head and body – and spent the rest of the afternoon cleaning up the mess made on the kitchen counter, mopping up the spilled sugar and rice and beans.

That was because everything stored away in the tins, fell out the moment they hit the counters. So another useful tip – make sure that all your tins are closed properly, and are fully air – tight, before you store them away your kitchen shelves and counters.

Do not put glass bottles on shelves high up. That is because unless the shelves are very steady, there is always a chance of an overladen shelf giving way. And broken glass all over your kitchen is not something conducive to safety.

Kitchen Furnishings

Call it a bit of childishness, but I cannot walk into my mother's gleaming kitchen without shuddering at her rows and rows of shining shelves made out of glass. And on each dainty shelf are lots and lots of glass bottles.

Even though the shelves have done their storing duty nobly for the past 30 years and more, I would not touch them or even approach them, because I am always very chary about glass furnishings in the kitchen. Just my point of view – I prefer my fixtures to be unbreakable.

You may want gleaming glass fixtures in the shape of shelves, to give your kitchen lots of elegance. But I prefer sturdy wood, well drilled into the wall and supported with lots of strong supports.

Your Kitchen Medical Cabinet

Remember to have these items ready at hand in your kitchen medicine cabinet. A good pair of scissors, pieces of lint and gauze, bandages, burn ointment, witch hazel, cotton wool, a good antiseptic and any soothing natural, healthy healing item like honey.

Knocks, sprains, dislocations, and other body injuries can be treated well, with witch hazel. Cuts and wounds should be treated with disinfectant. Call the doctor, if the cut are deep or have been caused by broken glass.

Clean the cut out well with boiling water, salt water and even Marigold water. If the bleeding does not stop, sprinkle the cut with lemon juice. My grandmother used some solid sugar on cut fingers in order to clot the blood.

If the cut is deep or inflamed, make an antiseptic soak with 6 drops of lavender oil, added to 1 cup of water. Soak the cut for at least 10 minutes, then apply honey or Marigold cream and cover with a clean bandage.

If you do not have lavender oil around, you can use a soak made up of water and Marigold petals.

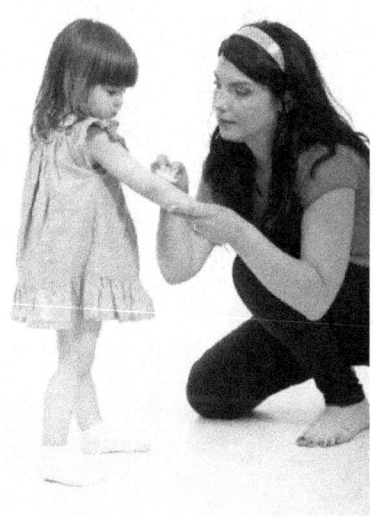

Suspected sprains, fractures, and dislocations will need the help of experienced doctors, so do not try to set them straight yourself.

Like I said before, you can place honey on a burn to prevent it from getting infected, before you can get to a doctor.

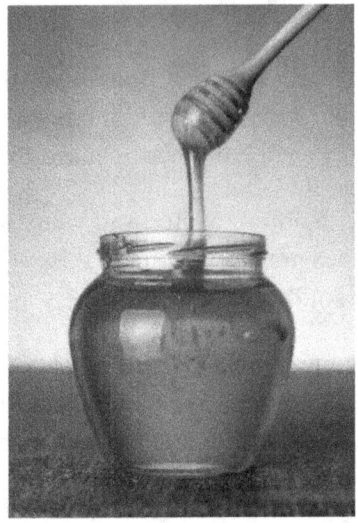

Honey is the best natural healer known to mankind.

Electric Accidents

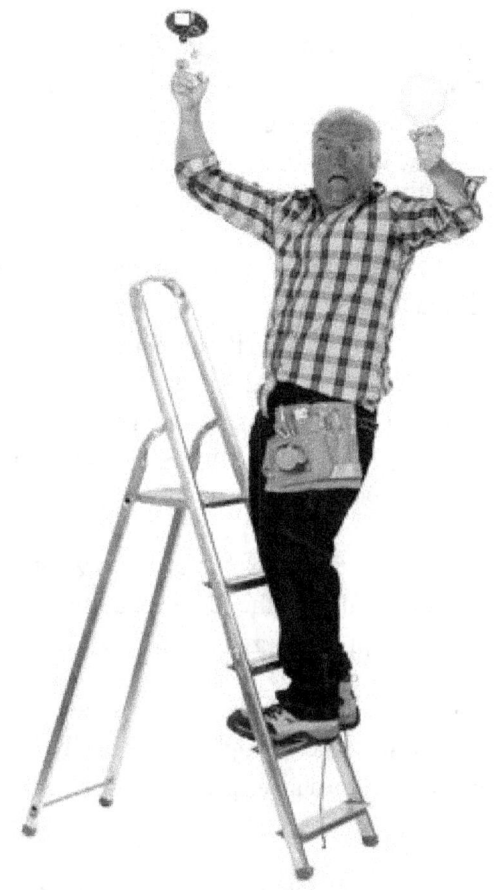

Do not let this happen, ever by being careless around electricity.

Thanks to the usage of so many electric gadgets in the kitchen, there is a chance of electric accidents, so you need to take these elementary precautions before you use them.

Never touch any electrical appliance with wet hands. Also, make sure that the floor is not wet, especially if you are barefoot. You may laugh and say, barefoot in the kitchen, and say something about savages, but believe it or not, many children enjoy walking barefoot, and if they walk into a kitchen, where the electric supply is not properly grounded and safe and the floor is wet, there is a chance of an electric accident occurring.

Also make sure that all the sockets in the kitchen walls are properly secure and away from the reach of children. Especially if you have a crawling baby in the house. A crawling baby goes directly to the nearest socket in the wall, even if it is not in the kitchen and if it is not baby proofed with electric plug guards, baby is going to get a tremendous shock.

There was one instance where my 10-month-old nephew – who had just begun to crawl – decided to stalk a cockroach across the floor. The triumphant hunter behind it and the terrified cockroach scuttling away from that little dynamo, away they went. Until they came up against a wall. And the baby forgot all about cockroaches as potentially amusing things with which to play the moment he saw the wall socket, right in front of his little nose.

This was something nice and new to explore, and in went his little fingers into the holes in the socket. Luckily they had plug guards on them and we hauled him away from it, he protesting vigorously.

However, in many cases, accidents do happen, because the sockets are not well grounded. So any wall socket, which can be easily accessible to children and toddlers should be totally safe, grounded and adventurous – baby- proofed.

Do not use any appliances with broken plugs or sockets or damaged flex. I have seen many appliances in many kitchens all over the world, with the covering over the flex damaging to the passing of time. You can see the colored wires exposed, and even though I tell the owners that this makes the appliance a potential kitchen hazard, the answer is – "hey, the electric wire is totally insulated with its plastic covering, is not it. So we are not worrying, we have been using this implement for the past umpteen years and it has not given us any trouble, so stop acting so paranoid."

The world is made up of people who will not learn or will just act stubborn, just because someone told them not to do something or cautioned them against something else.

These are the people who suffer from accidents, – including kitchen accidents – which they are definitely going to blame on their appliances, some manufacturing defects and other factors, but definitely not their own carelessness. Do not be one of them because your health and safety lies in your own hands.

Electricity needs to be treated with respect, in any form. Do not use any appliance whose plug is making a sizzling noise. That means there is some short-circuit in the wiring. In the same manner, if you plug in something in a wall socket, and there is an electrical spark, you need to call in an electrician or an experienced handyman to check the wiring.

Sizzling sounds mean loose wire connections, potential shocks to anybody using any electric appliance and even short circuits, which are going to blow out the wiring system in your kitchen.

Make sure to disconnect coffee percolator s or electric kettles before either filling or emptying them. Many half – asleep people making their early cup of Java are shocked awake, when they start emptying the hot liquid out in their cups, without switching off the electric kettle. In the same way, many accidents are caused when people forget is that they have switched on their electric kettle and start filling it with water. Best way to suffer an electric accident.

In the same way, if you are thinking of cleaning your electric range with soapy water and a cleaning cloth, remember to switch it off and remove the electric plug if any.

In case of any sort of electrical accidents in the kitchen or in the house, switch off the power supply immediately and call for professional medical help.

Gas Leaks

There have been many cases when people lit their gas burners, even when there was a slight smell of gas leaking in the kitchen. Always trace the leak, when there is the smell of gas and do not rest until the source has been found. It could be a loose gas hose connection or a faulty tap.

Also, use some common sense. Do not try looking for faulty connections with a candle. Someone told me that an acquaintance of his had done it, because being a mining engineer, they looked for the presence of methane and other inflammable gases in enclosed spaces with the help of a small, contained flame.

That does not work for gas, and is the best way in which you can help in the blowing up of your kitchen. That stubborn and I – Know – Best mining engineer did exactly that, using a lit candle and now he rests In Peace. I will not be a ghoul and Say I Told You so.

If the gas escape cannot be explained, get help as soon as possible by ringing up the Gas Company or agency. They are going to send a professional person immediately who is going to check the gas leak with soapy water. It is his job to deal with any case of leaking gas and replace any faulty parts in your gas range, if present. These could include the rubber gas tube or a leakage in the burners.

Accidental Poisoning

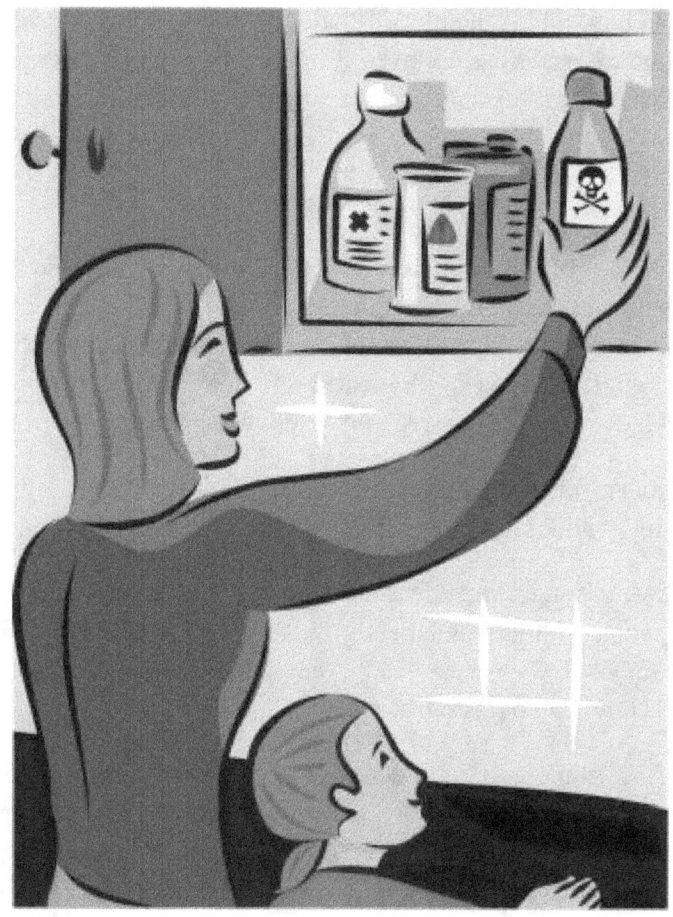

Most of the kitchens do double duty as cleaning places as well as cooking places. This is a place where you store your cleaning fluids, disinfectants and bleaches, which are powerful cleaning agents kept in the kitchen often most misleadingly in things like squash bottles or empty tomato sauce bottles.

Remember to label a cleaning fluid, if you are shifting it from its original container into one of these bottles. Suspect everything in the kitchen which you have not placed, in its rightful place.

My father has this bad habit of placing a powerful liquid insecticide in a bottle, right in my kitchen cabinet where I store other edible liquids. According to him, that is the place where he remembers he has kept that particular liquid. And he is annoyed if I place it away in a safer place, because he cannot get his hands on it really fast when he needs it.

All right, his logic is justified. But placing a poison where you are keeping your edible things is definitely not a sensible idea.

If you have a family member like father in your family, who likes things his own way, stop arguing. The best thing to do is to give that particular bottle a whole corner to itself with absolutely nothing around it or touching it. It is also labeled with a number of piratical skulls and crossbones in red and black, so that even the half asleep person knows that it is dangerous.

Remember to sniff anything doubtful, especially if it is in liquid form and you are going to add it to your cooking.

In the same way, some saltpeter crystals were placed in my spices cabinet and stayed there, without any labeling. Some years later, I took them out. What were they? Soda bicarbonate? They did not look like monosodium glutamate. They did not taste like salt.

Now my first mistake was that I did not label them before storing them away. Also, I had placed them in a place, where I normally kept my edible spices. That was mistake number 2. So remember, when you are putting away things which are of a potentially harmful nature in your kitchen cabinet, make sure that they are placed away from edible things.

Because a couple of years later, you may find yourself wondering whether it was powdered rat poison or what, and what was it doing in a spice cabinet, unlabeled and wrapped up in a cellophane paper?

Keep everything in the right place, and in the right container.

I remember going to a favorite aunt's house, and hunting for cookies. "Oh", she said insouciantly. "You are going to find them in the tin labeled Tea."

Now why would she want to put her cookies in the tin labeled "tea"? "Because I have them with tea," she explained.

Now that is some sort of logic which seems sensible to her, but which leaves me totally perplexed. I, being a more methodical person have salt in tins labeled "salt" and rice in tins labeled "rice".

That saves me and anybody else coming into the kitchen, plenty of wear and tear to your temper and nerves, especially when you know that you will not find cookies in tins labeled tea.

Also, it means that I am not going to have anything potentially dangerous floating around my shelves, in its unlabeled form, especially if it is a cleaning fluid, disinfectant and bleach.

These items should never be placed near edibles. Place them in storage areas under your kitchen sink.

If you get poisoned accidentally, seek professional help immediately. Remember to take the suspect substance along with you so that your doctor knows exactly how to treat the patient without wondering what could have caused that rising

For food poisoning, tried to induce vomiting by sticking your finger down the patient's throat. You can also give him an emetic drink made with one tablespoonful each of mustard powder and salt in a glassful of warm water.

Do not use emetics for poisoning by chemicals as you could make the situation worse.

Conclusion

Most accidents happen in your home, including your kitchen, just because you have not taken some elementary precautions. So the first rule of preventing such accidents from happening is by making your kitchen and your home as safe as possible. This is doubly necessary if there are children or old people about.

Make sure that medicines and household cleaning products are kept out of the reach of children and pets.

Look around your kitchen and home for other potentially dangerous areas. Use the electric plug guards.

Disorder, haste, carelessness and panic are some important factors which cause accidents. A clean and tidy kitchen with a level headed cook working in it is as safe as it can be.

Have a good smoke alarm installed in your kitchen. You may also want to attend a good first aid class, to know more how you can keep your family safe. Learn how you can use simple techniques for dealing effectively with household emergencies including kitchen accidents.

If an accident does occur, do not panic! Just stop, take deep, calming breaths, so that you can act more effectively and either call for help or contain the situation yourself, if you can do so.

Live Long and Prosper!

Author Bio

Dueep Jyot Singh is a Management and IT Professional who managed to gather Postgraduate qualifications in Management and English and Degrees in Science, French and Education while pursuing different enjoyable career options like being an hospital administrator, IT,SEO and HRD Database Manager/ trainer, movie , radio and TV scriptwriter, theatre artiste and public speaker, lecturer in French, Marketing and Advertising, ex-Editor of Hearts On Fire (now known as Solstice) Books Missouri USA, advice columnist and cartoonist, publisher and Aviation School trainer, ex-moderator on Medico.in, banker, student councilor ,travelogue writer … among other things!

One fine morning, she decided that she had enough of killing herself by Degrees and went back to her first love -- writing. It's more enjoyable! She already has 48 published academic and 14 fiction- in- different- genre books under her belt.

When she is not designing websites or making Graphic design illustrations for clients , she is browsing through old bookshops hunting for treasures, of which she has an enviable collection – including R.L. Stevenson, O.Henry, Dornford Yates, Maurice Walsh, De Maupassant, Victor Hugo, Sapper, C.N. Williamson, "Bartimeus" and the crown of her collection- Dickens "The Old Curiosity Shop," and so on… Just call her "Renaissance Woman") - collecting herbal remedies, acting like Universal Helping Hand/Agony Aunt, or escaping to her dear mountains for a bit of exploring, collecting herbs and plants and trekking.

Our books are available at

1. Amazon.com
2. Barnes and Noble
3. Itunes
4. Kobo
5. Smashwords
6. Google Play Books

Check out some of the other JD-Biz Publishing books
Gardening Series on Amazon

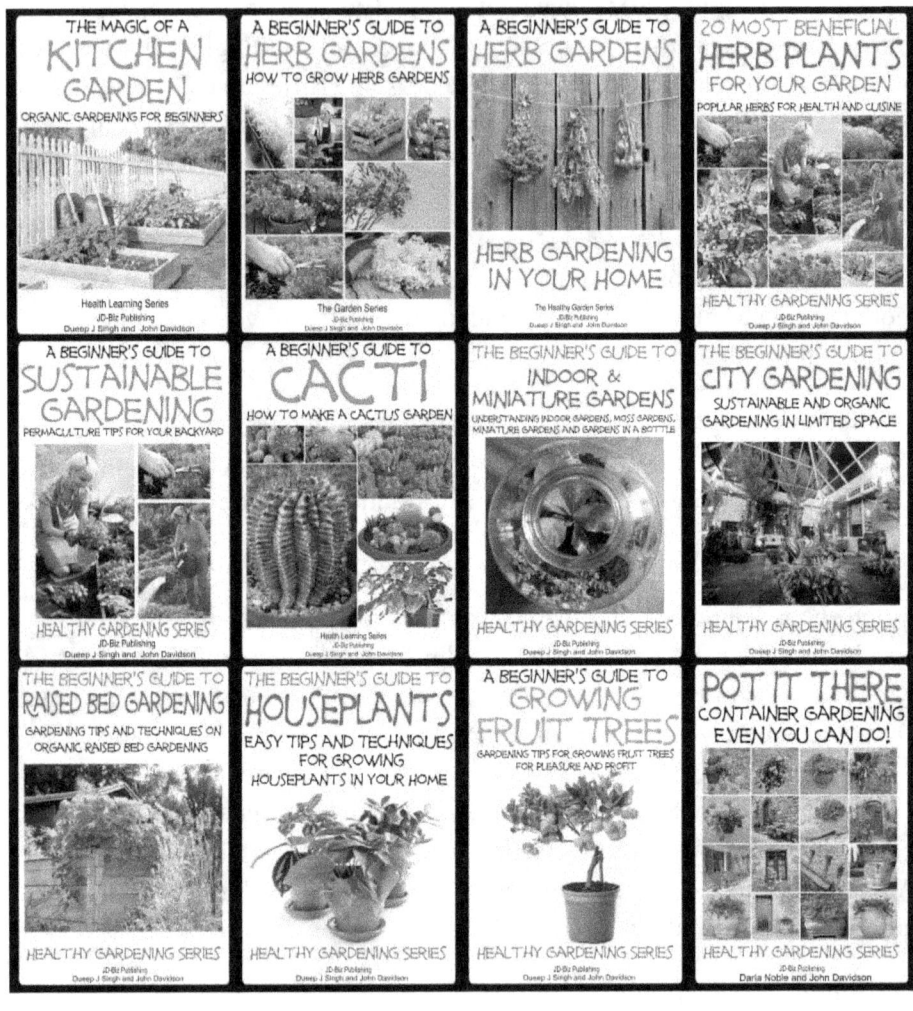

Health Learning Series

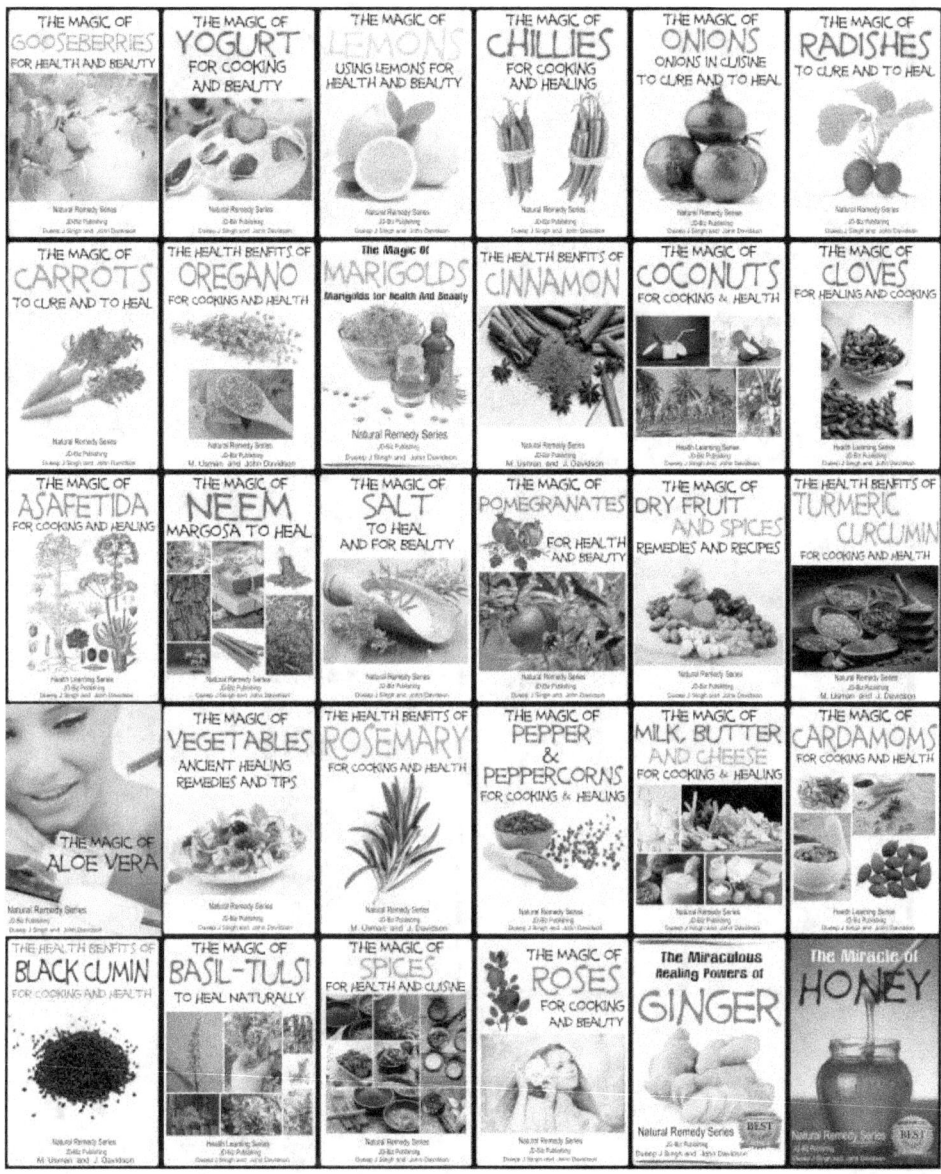

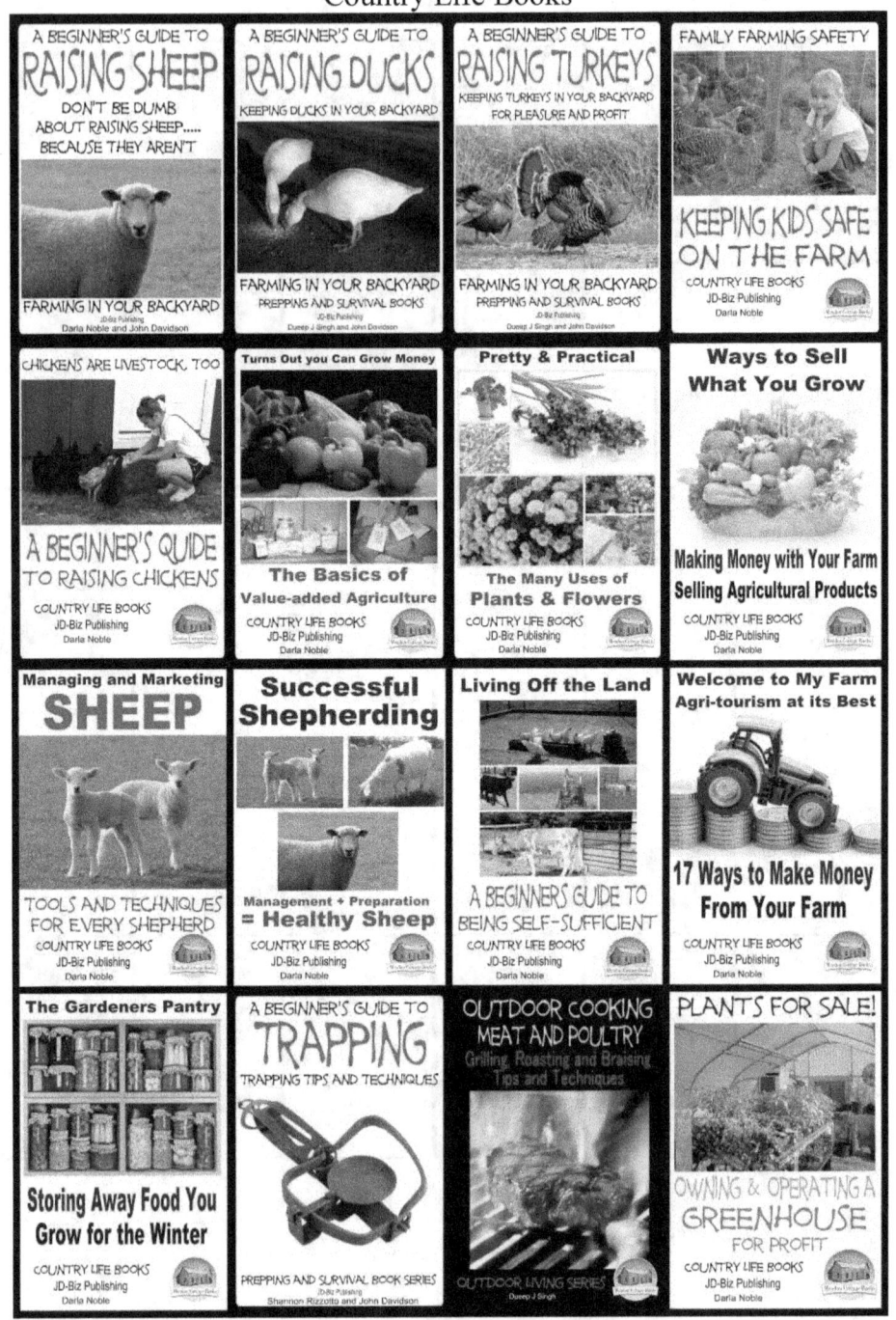

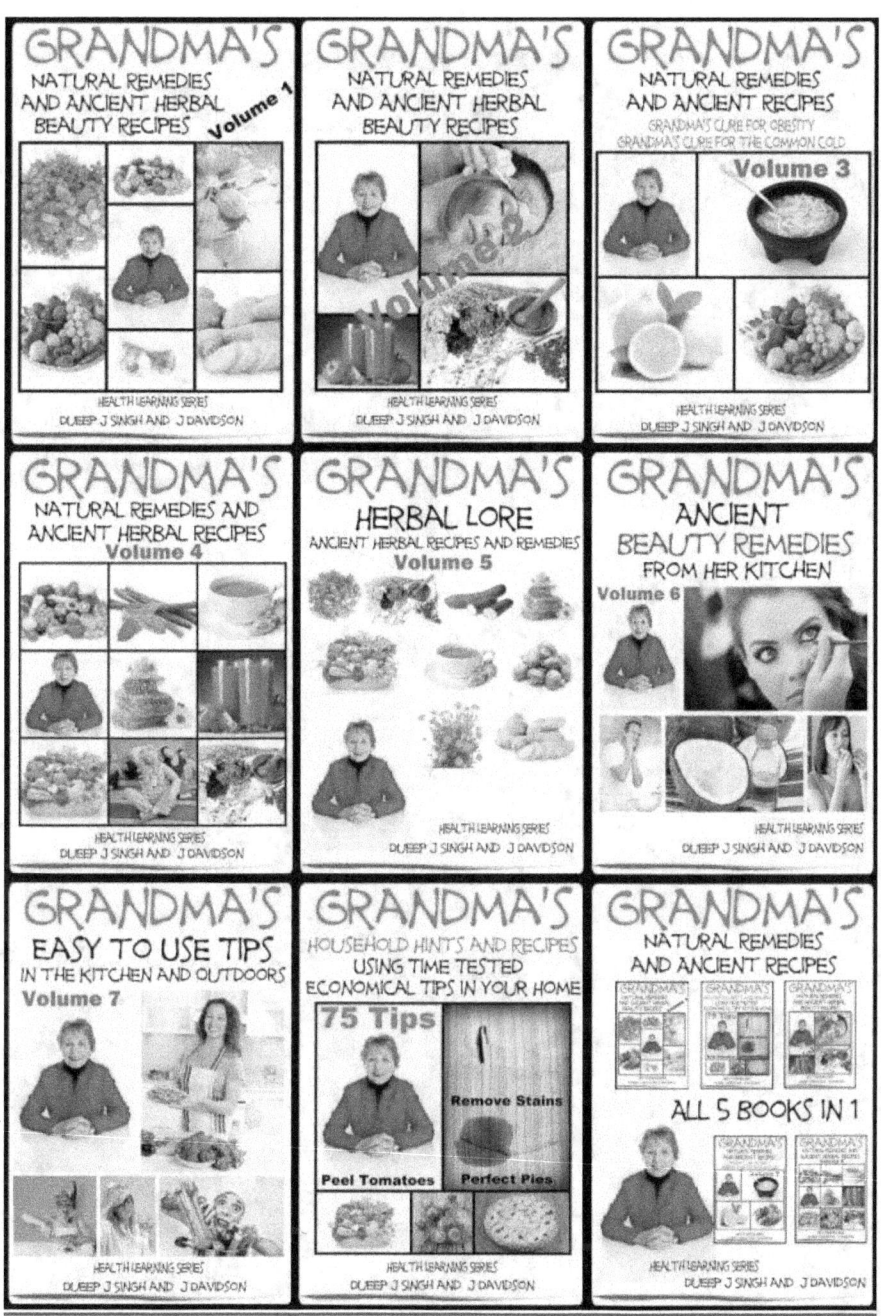

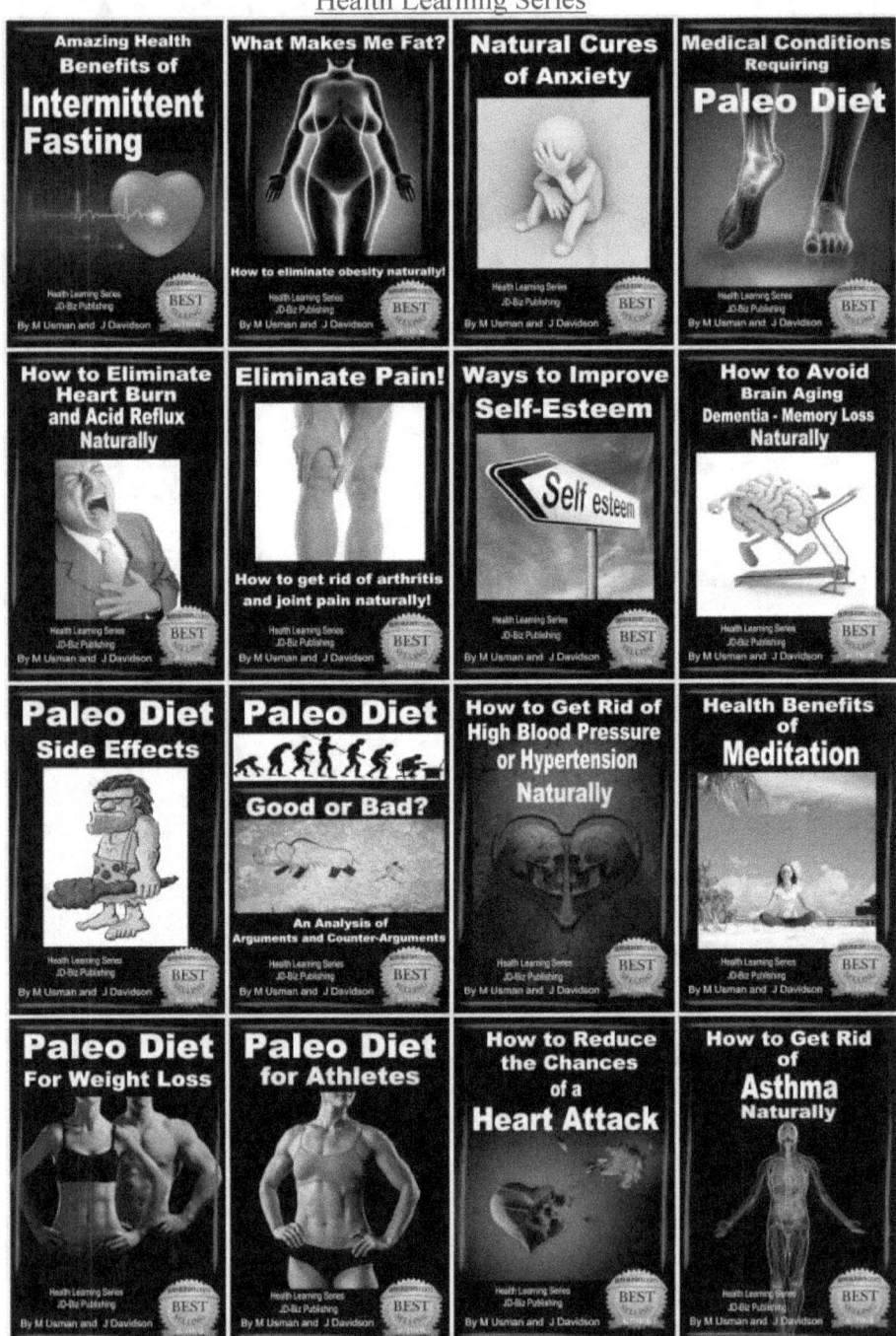

Amazing Animal Book Series

Chinchillas	Beavers	Snakes
Dolphins	Wolves	Walruses
Polar Bears	Turtles	Bees
Frogs	Horses	Monkeys
Dinosaurs	Sharks	Whales
Spiders	Big Cats	Big Mammals of Yellowstone
Animals of Australia	Sasquatch - Yeti Abominable Snowman Bigfoot	Giant Panda Bears
Kittens	Komodo Dragons	Lady Bugs
Animals of North America	Meerkats	Birds of North America
Penguins	Hamsters	Elephants

Learn To Draw Series

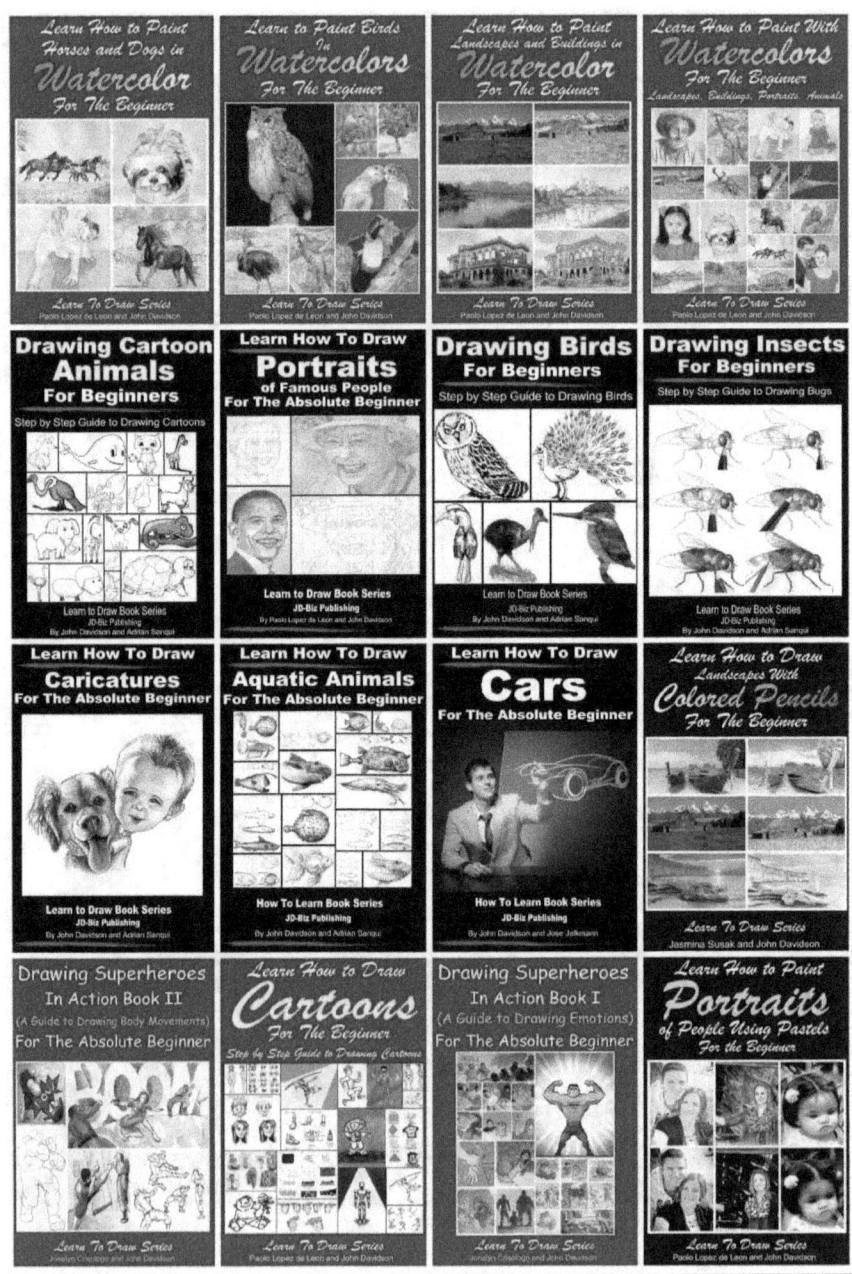

Entrepreneur Book Series

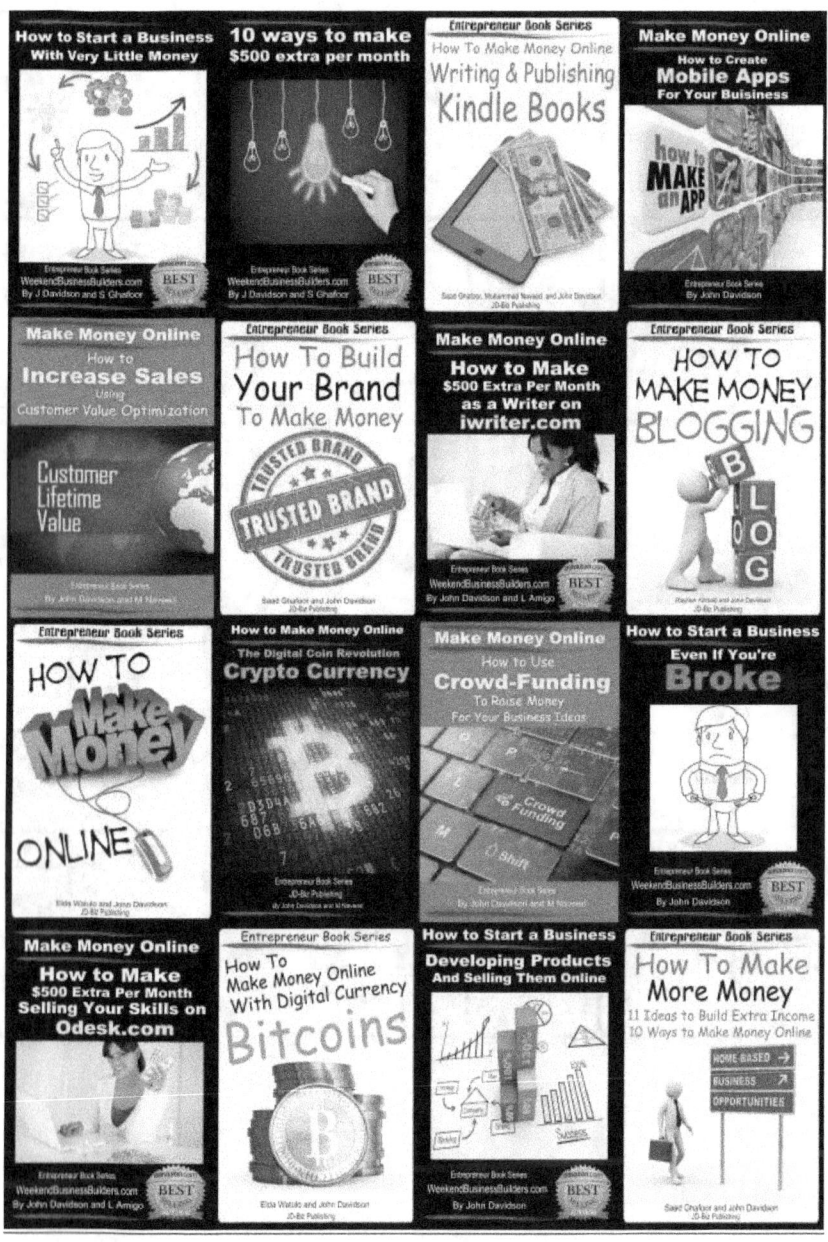

How to Build and Plan Books

Kitchen Safety – Tips to Prevent Kitchen Accidents

Publisher

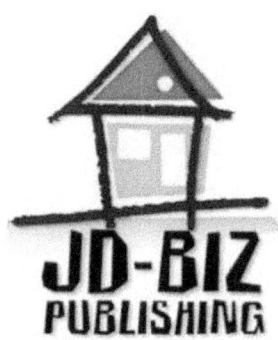

JD-Biz Corp

P O Box 374

Mendon, Utah 84325

http://www.jd-biz.com/

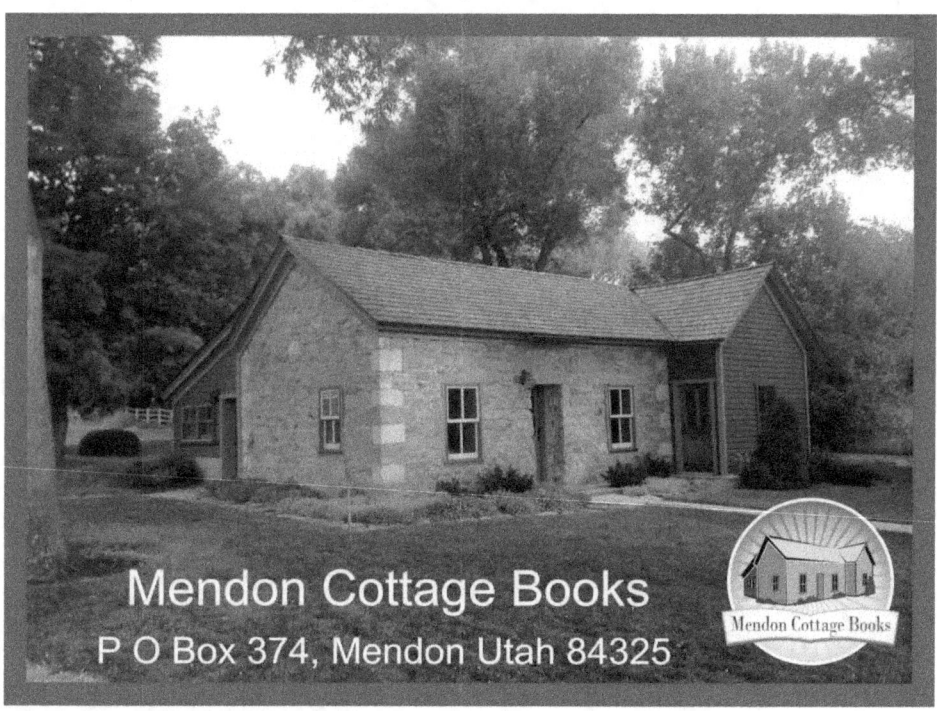

Mendon Cottage Books

P O Box 374, Mendon Utah 84325

www.ingramcontent.com/pod-product-compliance
Lightning Source LLC
Chambersburg PA
CBHW072018290526
45787CB00013B/1329